To: Charles McGrath

Enjoy the book!

Keeping the faith!

Donna M. Weston

Dedication

This book is dedicated to my loving husband Norris, and my two beautiful children Norissa and Norris IV, whose unyielding love and support was with me from day one of the rebirth and before.

THE RE-BIRTH

Memoirs of a Stem Cell Transplant

ISBN: 0-9710960-0-7

Blue Skies Publishing
P.O. Box 969
New York, New York 10027
(646) 698-0941

THE
RE-BIRTH
Memoirs of a Stem Cell Transplant

By
Donna M. Weston

Blue Skies Publishing
New York, New York

Acknowledgements

Thanks to everyone who supported me during the writing of this book. I could not have done it without your love and support, and you know who you are. Thanks to Wendy Grace Thorpe-Cruz who made sure I dotted my "i"s and crossed my "t"s. Thank you also to Teresa and Maria for their help.

TABLE OF CONTENTS

PROLOGUE

❖❖❖❖

Imagine being a young woman, thirty something years of age, married, with two children, a relatively nice job, and a letter of acceptance to an Ivy League graduate school program. Yes, I am ready. I have my spirituality in focus, the love and support of my family, and I am ready to take on the world. I am energized and poised for further success. Then one day, out of the clear blue sky, I noticed what appeared to be a breast deformity. The shape of my left breast had actually changed. I thought this phenomenon to be strange, but was not alarmed because I was getting regular check-ups and cancer screenings, and all had been well in the land of health (so I thought).

I marched myself up to the nearest cancer-screening clinic to have the breast checked out. After about three weeks, 1 mammogram, a muscle tissue biopsy, and a CAT scan, I was diagnosed with infiltrating ductal cell carcinoma – stage IIIB. Upon receiving immediate treatment of chemotherapy, which was not effective, I underwent a modified radical mastectomy. A few months later, my doctors urged me to undergo a peripheral stem-cell transplant (also referred to as an autologous bone marrow transplant) in conjunction with high dose chemotherapy. In this procedure, according to the American Cancer Society, bone marrow or stem cells from the blood are taken from the patient and reinfused after high doses of chemotherapy have been administered. The treatment is commonly used in women with advanced breast cancer, but there is a growing trend for its use in patients with earlier stages of breast cancer. Also, according to the American Cancer Society, cancer is the second largest cause of death in the United States, exceeded only by heart disease. Cancer does not discriminate. It ignores one's race, ethnicity, religious background, age, and sexual orientation. You need not even be of the human species to develop cancer.

Because autologous bone marrow, and peripheral stem cell transplants are relatively new procedures, conclusive success rate statistics are not yet available. According to my doctor, there is approximately an eighty-five percent success rate. My doctors tell me that the benefits outweigh the side effects. I am hoping that is the case for me. My surgeon told me that I had a 5 to 10 percent chance of surviving 5 years after the transplant. It would take all that I had mentally, physically, and spiritually, to endure what happened next.

The pages in this book will reflect a psychological account of a twenty-three day medical procedure, written from the perspective of me, the patient. The accounts are both during, and retrospective of, my physiological ordeal. While revisiting and analyzing my hospital stay, I decided to incorporate my personal thoughts in the forms of poetry and prose, or what I call, "*ponderances of the day*", to sum up my feelings as each day passed. I hope you will find them to be insightful, inspirational, and amusing. I wrote them all.

This book is also for anyone who has either had cancer, presently has cancer, knows someone who has or had it, or who has an interest in knowing what it might be like to undergo a peripheral stem-cell transplant in conjunction with high dose chemotherapy.

This book should serve as a source of inspiration and hope for a bright future for people with advanced stages of cancer. It is conquerable and I plan to conquer it, fully. The readers of this book of memoirs should understand that the rebirth that unfolds within these pages is truly a rebirth in every sense of the word. It is a rebirth of the body, mind, and spirit. And, as with any rebirth, the offspring comes back into life's forces with renewed hope, spirit and endless possibilities. I wish you success in your rebirth should you choose to undergo one. May the spiritual forces bestow their unyielding healing and existential powers upon you. Please have every reason to feel positive, confident, and empowered with a sense of self-actualization and hope that only a divine consummation can achieve.

Keeping the faith,

Donna M. Weston

THE DAY BEFORE

❖❖❖❖

Today was a fun-filled day. I had an appointment to have some stitches removed from a port and catheter that had been taken out due to infection seventeen days prior. I was rushed to St. Luke's hospital in New York City, where I endured a ten-day stay on intravenous anti-biotics. It had not been fun, and needless to say, I had not looked my best. I would be meeting with the surgeon who removed the port for the first time as an outpatient. I purchased a new wig, robed a cool lime green dress draped with a soft, pleasantly coordinated scarf. I felt like a diva and received the attention of one the whole day.

As I arrived at the receptionist's desk area of the doctor's office and began to sign in, the surgeon stepped over to the desk with his head buried deep into a patient file he had been perusing. For a moment, the doctor looked up and our eyes met. His perplexed look told me he had not recognized me. When I smiled and said hello, he knew who I was. What a difference a dress and a wig can make!

My daughter was scheduled to participate in a talent show at her day care center. She was very concerned about whether or not I would show up since I missed a few of her earlier shows due to illness and work commitments. I was determined to make her happy by showing up promptly. When I arrived on time and sat in the front row of the room, my daughter's head protruded from behind the makeshift curtains with the biggest smile I had ever seen on her face. She called out to me and waved her hand, verifying her satisfaction and relief that her mother had indeed showed up. Shortly thereafter, my husband arrived. We watched the show, had cookies and refreshments and headed home afterwards.

When we arrived home, I checked the messages on the answering machine as I had always done. There was a message from a New York Hospital representative who stated I should report to the admissions office at 11:00 a.m. the next day. That night, sleep did not come easy as I contemplated what the future might hold for me, and whether I would even have a future. Also that night, as my family laid in a peaceful slumber, I watched over them. Although I had done that many times before, that night it was different because I did not know if I would get the chance to do it again. It was a long night of mixed emotions.

DAY ONE

❖❖❖❖

It is 11:00 a.m. and I arrive promptly at The New York Hospital – Cornell Medical Center admissions office. I proceed to the reception area where I am warmly greeted, and obviously expected. I am asked to have a seat and, I do so quietly. A few moments later a phone rings and the receptionist answers it. "Yes she is here, she just arrived at 11:00 a.m.", she replies after a moment of silence. I was the only one in the waiting room and thought gee- they sure are anxious to have me here. The room was pleasant and the atmosphere relaxing. The receptionist stepped out momentarily and when she returned, she informed me that my bed was ready. I smiled and thought to myself, great! I waited for about forty-five minutes before I was called into the back office to give my insurance information and receive my identification bracelet.

I was escorted upstairs to my room where I was greeted by a welcoming group of registered nurses. I met the nursing crew and a team of doctors. They assured me that they would take good care of me, but were divorced of any surety that I would be all right. I was extremely apprehensive about the whole idea of stem cell transplant but considered the possible alternative, and decided not to walk out of the hospital at that moment. I sat by the window and stared out of it for hours. It was very quiet in the room and in the hospital wing. After what seemed like an eternity, I as able to relax amidst the solitude.

I received a new catheter that night, which proved to be annoying because two young residents had difficulty reaching the vein successfully. After repeated attempts to permeate the vein, a victory was won! I was relieved, and rested comfortably in anticipation of the next day's events. My husband and children stopped by. I sensed an air of support from my family members. We knew that the upcoming physiological challenges would be great. Mentally I note that my children are very active, and will need something to occupy their time while on hospital visits. The family left at about 10:00p.m., and I went to sleep for the night. The next few weeks will prove to be the most challenging few weeks of my life.

❖❖❖❖

We know not what tomorrow brings;
Yet, each day, a mockingbird sings;
Like the songs in our hearts that speak new things;
What if we too had wings?

❖❖❖❖

DAY TWO

❖❖❖❖

The high dose chemotherapy (chemo) starts today. After a series of blood, urine and anal cultures, I am primed with sodium potassium in order to hydrate my system. Shortly thereafter the chemo is connected to my intravenous line. There are 3 types – cyclophosphamide, Thiotepa, and Carboplatin. The chemotherapies will totally destroy the bone marrow, placing me at risk of infection and bleeding. The period of risk will last 3 to 5 weeks until my previously stored stem cells are replaced into my body and begin to grow normally. Some possible side effects are nausea, vomiting; lowering of blood counts which could cause fatigue; bladder irritation; sterility; heart muscle damage; mouth sores; diarrhea; leukemia; loss of appetite; dizziness; headache; irregularities in menstrual cycle; skin rash; hives; decreased heart pumping functions, muscle weakness and hearing loss. In most instances, the chances of experiencing many of these side effects are minute. The largest complaints from peripheral stem cell/bone marrow transplant patients are nausea, fatigue, headache, and in my case, an overwhelming sense of restlessness.

Today is not a bad day because the chemo is slowly dripped around the clock and anti-nausea medication is abundantly administered. I ate breakfast, lunch and dinner and found it to be quite enjoyable. I felt no nausea today. My vital signs are checked regularly around the clock and the staff is caring, responsive, and efficient. I doze off to sleep at about 11:00p.m.

❖❖❖❖

Anticipation is like a rock;
It's hard to those who are hit with it;
And we must co-exist with it on this earth forever.

❖❖❖❖

DAY THREE

❖❖❖❖

The chemo is still going for the second day (remember, I did not start the chemo until the day 2). I am still in generally good spirits and am able to eat my breakfast, lunch and dinner. I walk around the unit floor a bit with my entourage of intravenous lines. I now begin to realize that a big problem will be boredom. I stroll back to my room to watch television. The hospital only has basic cable so I am limited to what I can watch. My television routine will likely consist of the local morning news show, various talk shows, some comedy shows (it helps to laugh), a few public access stations and the CNN news channel.

I spend the day receiving phone calls from family and friends, and switching from bed to chair and back again. My window is located on the side of the front entrance of the hospital building. I watch the people as they drive and walk to and from the main entrance doors. There is a pretty patch of foliage amidst the busy driveway area that offers some relief from the four walls of my hospital room. My mother comes in to visit me. She takes a handful of the rubber gloves that must be donned before entering my room. She claims they are great for administering hair color. My mother's action embarrasses me and I think to myself, I'm glad there is nothing else she can take from the hospital room that can be carried in her purse. Mother and I watch television together and spend the day talking. My husband and the children arrive later. The children are restless and prove to be my next source of embarrassment by running around from the bathroom to the lounge and back reeking havoc by fighting over trivial issues. You gotta love it! We talk, watch television, listen to the children argue back and forth, and the family leaves for the night. I watch a little more television, and try to fall asleep.

❖❖❖❖

I once saw a woman with a toddler
caught in a storm, with no umbrella;
I, while 8 months pregnant,
offered them mine;
I hope God remembers.

❖❖❖❖

DAY FOUR

❖❖❖❖

Today is the third day of high dose chemo. I am beginning to experience the nausea associated with the procedure. There is a blue chair next to my bed that emits a foul odor. I cannot quite describe the smell, but it reminds me of the chemo. My nausea increases whenever I smell the chair. It is very annoying, but I forget to tell the nurses and doctors when they come in for progress checks. It is becoming more difficult to sit at the window due to the smell of the "stinky" chair. My breakfast arrives and I have no desire to eat it. I have been using an anti-bacterial mouth rinse to help prevent mouth sores. The rinse is beginning to nauseate me. I am supposed to use it every four hours but it is becoming increasingly difficult to do so. I begin to vomit. The vomiting is brought on by the heparin and saline flushes used to clean my catheter lines. The vomit taste like medicine and it is very troublesome. I proceed to vomit about 3 more times within a 6-hour period. I try to watch television but focusing and concentrating becomes a challenge. I can tell that the chemo is affecting my brain. I began to feel heaviness in my chest area during my previous hospital stay (the result of a blood clot from the port). The chest heaviness is quite troublesome because it feels as though my heart and lungs are caving in. This sensation creates more nausea and stress and I find it necessary to incorporate relaxation techniques into my daily schedule. I feel weak and I am growing increasingly restless. I want this whole ordeal to be over soon. I am aware of every second that goes by. I try to fill my day with sleep. When night comes, I am restless. I go to the bathroom about 10 times. I am starting not to like this stem cell transplant very much, to say the least.

❖❖❖❖

Life is what we make it;
Love is what we give;
Trust is what we hope for;
Trust in your God,
It's how we should live.

❖❖❖❖

DAY FIVE

❖❖❖❖

Today is the fourth day of high dose chemo. This day is virtually a replica of yesterday. My day is filled with excessive vomiting with nothing to come up because I have not been eating. Television is becoming increasingly difficult to watch. It is hard to take my mind off of the situation that is staring me in the face. I turn to my gospel music. It uplifts my spirits. I try to focus on taking it one day at a time, but I am overwhelmingly bombarded with the feeling of restlessness. I do not know what to do with myself. I change positions in the bed from top to bottom. I try to sing but my voice is gone due to weakness. I pray. I sit in the "stinky" chair, but can only take it for a minute or two. I get back into bed. I toss and I turn. I pray again. I listen to the gospel music again. The phone rings but I do not answer it because I am void of the desire to speak to anyone. It continues to ring until I unplug it. I now feel guilty because I know that people are concerned about my situation and want to know how I am feeling. The guilt soon passes and I begin more prayer. I elect to keep the telephone unplugged. I have long conversations with God and ask him to show me a sign of whether or not I would successfully emerge from my medical ordeal. I immediately begin to feel a sense of assurance. I know that God is watching over me. Sleep does not come easy throughout the night. I am averaging about 3 hours of sleep per night. It is not helping my situation. I am growing increasingly irritable and frustrated. I just want to go home now. It is difficult to think of anything else. I am disconnected from the chemo at 1:00 a.m.

❖❖❖❖

I'm hungry, but I can't eat;
I'm sleepy, but I can't sleep;
I'm funny, but I can't laugh;
Heck, I can't even take a bath;
What am I gonna do all day?
I know. I'll pray.

❖❖❖❖

DAY SIX

❖❖❖❖

I awake from a sporadic sleep pattern, relieved that the chemo is no longer running through my intravenous line. Shortly thereafter I was disconnected from the hydration fluids. I would be free from my entourage of intravenous substances for two days. This process allows time for the chemo to be discarded from my system through urination. I am still nauseated, but the feeling of liberation has lessened the blow of the nausea. I sit on an ottoman and rest my head on the side of my bed with my arms cloaking a pillow. I listen to my gospel to no avail. There is a short in the wire and the sound keeps going in and out. I snatch off the earphones and throw the Walkman on the bed. I am now ready to lash out at the first person that walks through my hospital room door. Unfortunately, I do not have the strength to do it, and I quickly dismiss the thought. I don my rubber gloves and air-filtering mask and stroll through the corridors of my wing. Although I am tired, I realize the need to exercise to build my strength. I head back to my room, remove my protective gear and again sit in the "stinky" chair to look out of window. After a few moments, I get back into bed. I try to take a nap. I toss, turn, pray, and wish it would all soon be over.

Evening falls and my husband and the children arrive. I am always happy to see them. The children proceed with their usual trivial, yet, highly annoying quarreling matches. I try to ignore it, but it is difficult. I lack the momentum to intercede and reprimand them for their behavior. My husband senses that the children are becoming problematic and elects to leave for home. I become ambivalent because I really want to be with them, but my two little "stress factors" are tilting the stability equation right now, to say the least. The family left at about 10:00 p.m. and I tossed and turned until about 2:00 a.m. before I fell into a much needed slumber.

❖❖❖❖

Is my life in the hands of the doctors;
Who prescribe the medicine for me?
Or in the hands of the books I read;
That tells me which way to be?
Is it in the hands of the things I choose?
Do they determine whether I win or lose?
Do I sit back and let life play out for me?
I don't know, I guess I'll see.
Who is that speaking to me?
You say you want me to hear your plea;
To open up, and listen to thee;
That my life is in your hands, you say;
To that, I reply;
I'll be o.k.

❖❖❖❖

DAY SEVEN

❖❖❖❖

Today is my second "free" day. That is, a day without intravenous connection. The day is progressing relatively uneventfully with the exception of a few vomiting episodes. I am beginning to get used to the vomiting, so the incidents seem to pass without much stress. I am actually relieved of nausea momentarily, after vomiting. So strangely, it almost becomes a welcomed event. I walk around the unit a few times. I sit in the lounge that consists of a television, some chairs, and pamphlets regarding various medical issues. This lounge is not the most exciting place one could frequent. I stroll back to my room and proceed to watch television. I received a few visitors and phone calls. There really is not much to do but wait, and wait, and wait. The restlessness according to my doctor, is a good sign that the patient is doing relatively well. His rationale is that, if I am bored, there are probably not a lot of physical complications. So, in other words, the best case scenario is an extreme state of boredom. I really must practice using patience in order to keep my head leveled.

My little team of "angelic stress factors" arrives with my husband. We proceed with our tender moments of hugs and kisses, and shortly thereafter, they begin their trivial quarreling. I try to distance myself from the brother and sisterly love, but it is difficult. Now is a good time for deep breathing exercises, so I begin the process. In, and out. In, and out. The children join in. They calm down for a few seconds. And I do mean a few seconds. The family left after a few hours.

I begin to draw pictures today. I am severely challenged when I am faced with artistic drawing. I attempt to draw the entrance of the hospital, but when the drawing was completed, I could not tell what it was. I decide I should stick to writing. After more hours of television, I retire to bed at about 11:30 p.m. I say a prayer and off to sleep I go.

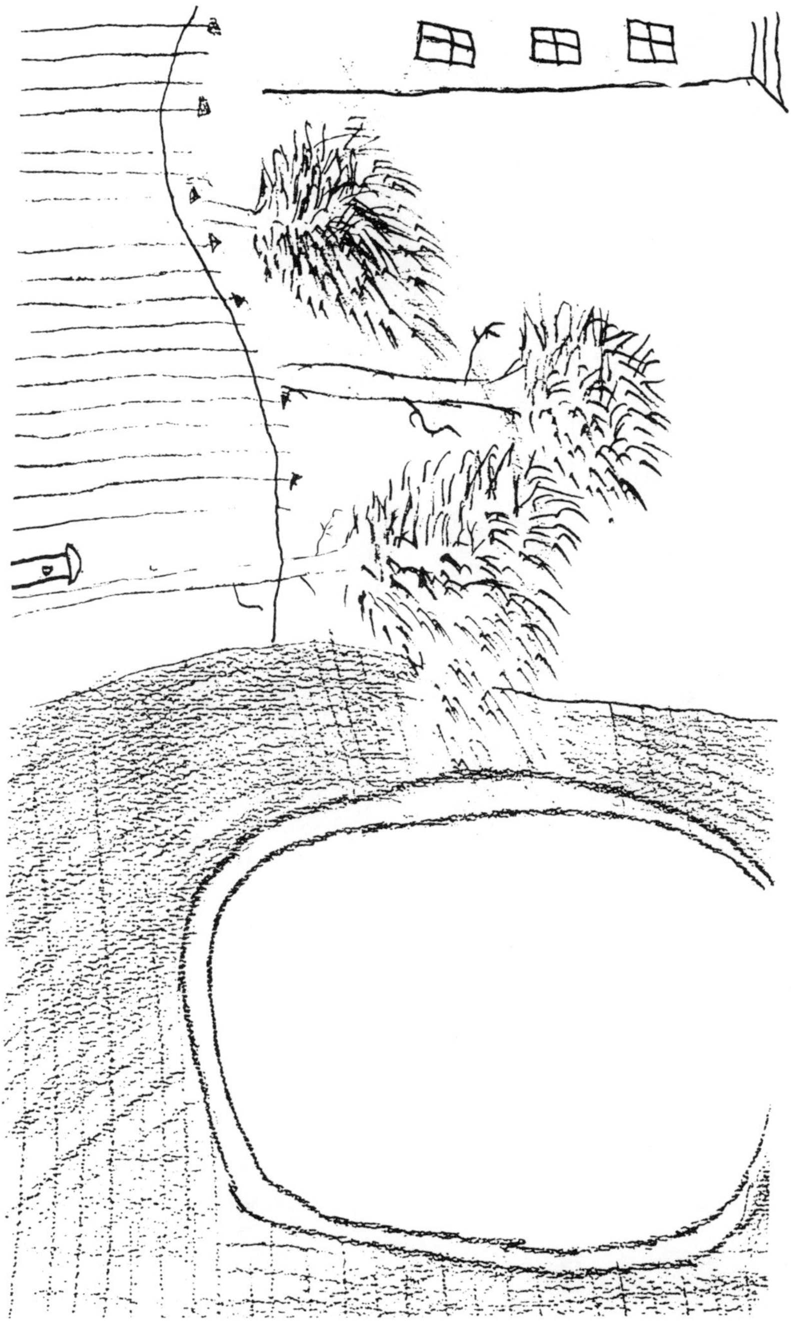

❖❖❖❖

When I was a little girl;
I wondered what I would be when I grew up.
I'm grown up now;
And I'm still wondering.

❖❖❖❖

DAY EIGHT

❖❖❖❖

Today I get hooked up to my entourage of intravenous antibiotics, and sodium chloride for hydration. It is annoying to have to make so many trips to the bathroom with the intravenous lines. It seems as though I have no place to turn for comfort from the nausea and the monotony. I again gaze out of the window as the people flow in and out of the hospital; and I picture the day that I will be among the "out-flowing". I listen to my "ocean sounds" relaxation music. It is very relaxing and it usually puts me to sleep. Unfortunately, I do not like sleeping during the day because I have such difficulty sleeping at night. I receive my daily slew of phone calls. I watch television for a few hours. My family visits again. I lie in bed most of the day. I count the days before I can leave. The doctors begin to hint at a longer than anticipated stay. I grow very annoyed because I was quoted 21 days and that is what I expected. I am beginning to question the validity of the statements of the doctors. I listen to my gospel music and pray to get home soon. I watch more television and eventually go to bed at about 11:00 p.m. My sleep is sporadic.

Throughout the night, as I toss and turn, I notice that my brain feels as though it is marinating. It is difficult to describe the feeling any better than previously stated. I would compare the feeling to that of the heat waves one sees from a large airplane exhaust system during take-off. It is as though my brain matter is boiling and the steam is rising from my head. The feeling is not painful, just different. I suppose it is my compromised equilibrium. This feeling, combined with the nausea is not a good thing.

❖❖❖❖

Here today;
Here tomorrow;
Hopefully...

❖❖❖❖

DAY NINE

❖❖❖❖

Today is the day I receive my stem cells back. I am so nervous that I can not stop shaking. I feel totally out of control. I do not know what to expect, and I am having difficulty calming myself down. I try my breathing technique but it offers no relief. The nurse comes in. She is both very patient and compassionate in assuring me that everything will be all right. She thoroughly explains the procedure (the transplant is done at my bedside). The procedure does not consist of much more than taking two Tylenol® tablets and a shot of Benadryl to prevent fever and allergic reaction to any preservatives that might have lingered in the stem cells (the preservatives are extracted before administering the stem cells to the patient).

As I am waiting, the minutes seem like hours. My stem cells arrive at about 11:00 a.m. I am somewhat calmed down from the Benadryl. The stem cells are connected to my intravenous lines and begin to flow through my veins. The process is painless. My level of fear was greatly outweighed by the procedure itself. Two hours passed and I am about three-quarters of the way finished with the treatment. When the transplant was completed, I vomited and got chills. I received Demerol, which calmed me down. After about two hours, I felt much better.

I am now waiting for my stem cells to engraft (join and begin to rebuild my immune system). The engraftment process usually takes about nine days, according to medical staff. Needless to say, I am counting down the days to engraftment completion. Once the required engraftment level has been met for twenty-four hours, a patient may go home provided no complications exist. I am more that ready for this to happen. I shall pray on it tonight.

❖❖❖❖

How can I express the way I feel;
Without shouting to the world, and pounding steal;
Without stomping my feet, and spitting the ground;
How can I smile, when I want to frown?
How can I laugh, when I want to cry?
How can I live, when I want to die?
How can I be strong, when I feel so weak?
How can I sing, when I can't even speak?
How, you ask, can you do these things?
Just take my hand, and spread your wings;
Come with me in flight, and as you soar;
These negative things will exist no more;
I can make your thoughts anew;
Just trust me, you'll see what I can do;
And when you've overcome your plight;
Take someone else's hand in flight;
Let them know it will be O.K.;
Just trust in me, that is the way.

❖❖❖❖

Note

❖❖❖❖

The next few days will be accounted for retrospectively because I was too weak to write. Although I maintained the mental capacity to be aware of, and to remember my surroundings, I lacked the momentum to detail it in writing. So, here it is…

❖❖❖❖

DAY TEN

❖❖❖❖

With the combination of a highly compromised immune system; various toxic medications; the stress of being in the hospital practically immobile for eleven days; not knowing what the outcome would be; and not receiving any real assurance that I would come out on top; I went into what I would call a state of delayed shock. Everything seemed surreal. It was as though my life was moving in slow motion, and nothing made much sense. All activities seemed to be taking place from a distance. I wanted to crawl under a rock and take up residency until I was better. I accepted no phone calls during that time. I was unable to concentrate on anything. I remember the psychological analyst coming in, and I asked her to please come back another time. This series of events indicated to me, that there was definitely something major going on inside of me. I could not eat. I do not think I ate the whole time I was there, other than the first two days. Most people have a tendency to gain weight from all the intravenous fluids they receive. I lost nineteen pounds. I could do nothing other than stare at the walls. It even became difficult to pray. I just waited out the time like a cocoon waiting to morph into a butterfly. A minute seemed like an hour. An hour seemed like a day. All I could think about was how long the whole ordeal would take to complete. I vaguely remember my family coming in to visit. I was not at all responsive to them. They basically sat around for as long as they could, then they left for home. Needless to say, these were not the best days of my life. And, this was one day I would have welcomed sleep.

In my nocturnal slumber I dreamed of being in a bombed out city looking for a way out. I was running through the back yards of partially standing buildings that led to dead ends. There was a man dressed in black, high above me, off in the distance, who appeared to be watching me. I repeatedly asked him if he knew the way out, but he never answered me. He just watched as I raced around like a rat in a maze looking for the cheese. Needless to say, that night's dream offered no solace from my monotonous reality.

❖❖❖❖

Time...
Some people spend it;
Some people waste it;
Some people clock it;
Others forsake it;
Some people know it;
Some people don't;
Some people cherish it;
Others just won't;
Some use it wisely;
Some not so smart;
Some say that time;
Should not keep us apart;
Others say time is just a big waste;
Those are the ones who use it in haste;
Time is a thing we should keep on our side;
A thing from which we can not hide;
We use our time with our own free will;
Just know that time;
Does not stand still.

❖❖❖❖

DAY ELEVEN

❖❖❖❖

On this day when I awoke, I was struck with a strange feeling I had from the vivid dream the night before. I was unable to shake that dream for some reason. I offered numerous analyses to myself and repeatedly concluded that literally, I was in a place I wanted to get out of, but was not sure of the exact method of breaking away. And, although people were around to help, they offered no real solutions to remedying my situation.

The day went on as a replica of the day before – filled with restlessness and a feeling of hopelessness. I tried to watch television but it served no real purpose. Today was a day that I skipped my shower against doctor's recommendation. "Let him take the damn shower," I said to myself. This uneventful day led to a series of thoughts and contemplations from, wondering if I would live through this whole ordeal, to, pondering why "stuff like this" happens to people who are trying to make a real positive difference in the world. I gleaned from my contemplations the enlightenment that there is a higher being with a specific purpose for each and every one of us, and that eventually, I would know my exact purpose. For now, it is to wait and get better.

That night, as I slept, I had another intense dream. The difference between the new dream and the last dream was that I recalled being in the second dreamland previously. I recognized the town and knew where certain landmarks were located. This town did not exist on earth, but I was very familiar with it. Although I was not previously acquainted with any of the town's people, they knew me. The town's people were having a meeting to decide whether or not they should allow me to leave town. The consensus was that I should stay forever, but I wanted to leave. Suddenly, I found myself in hiding. Everyone was looking for me everywhere. Finally, the town's people surrounded me and I began to talk them out of holding me hostage forever. I reasoned with them by pointing out the fact that it made no sense to keep me there against my will because I would not be a productive citizen. At that point, a path was opened for me and I was allowed to leave freely. Analysis: Perhaps if they had not let me go, I would never have come back to earth.

❖❖❖❖

When there's a will,
There's a way ***out****.*

❖❖❖❖

DAY TWELVE

❖❖❖❖

On this day I awoke to the reality that it was Independence Day. I immediately thought about the family outing I would be missing. It was somewhat depressing to know that I would be stuck in a hospital room while everyone else in the country would be celebrating. I then chose to focus on my health and decided that if I wanted to see another Independence Day, I should do whatever I could do, to make myself healthy.

I was extremely tired on this day and did not expect many visitors, in recognition of the upcoming events of the day. The day passed without many incidents. I tried to watch some television but could not really concentrate. I took a short walk along the corridor but became very tired, so I thought it best to stay near the bed. That night along the East River (which is where the hospital sits) fireworks would be displayed. I arranged to watch them from a window but was unable to do so when the time came. It seemed as though I stood too long in the shower and became extremely weak and could not watch the fireworks as a result. I remember falling back onto the bed and having absolutely no strength. It was the most overwhelming sense of weakness I had ever experienced. I really wanted to watch the fireworks but there was no way to make it happen. I just listened from my bed and said a few prayers. Needless to say, that was not the best Fourth of July for me.

❖❖❖❖

We never really know what dish
the chef of life will serve us;
we just drop in, mind the hot plate;
and hope it tastes good.

❖❖❖❖

DAY THIRTEEN

❖❖❖❖

Today is the day after Independence Day and all is relatively quiet. I was unbelievably weak last night and I am relieved to be feeling stronger today. I go through my daily routine of doctors' visits and blood analysis. I realize that I am passed the mid-way point in my hospital stay. I still cannot think of anything other than going home. I talk on the phone for awhile, watch television, and try to read. I can not help feeling that I am in a prison and my illness and intravenous lines are the bars that keep me from escaping. I cannot wait to be free!

My tenacious family makes their daily visit. I do not seem to have much to say lately. I think that this is the longest period of silence I have endured since being in my mother's womb. This whole medical process really is like a rebirth; because everything inside my immune system gets broken down to nearly nothing, and then begins to build up all over again. It is similar to the way an embryo starts out as a few cells, and then grows into a different and complete entity. My family gives the description of the festivities of the prior day. I listened from a mental distance, and tried to seem interested. Sometimes I wish I could jump out of my skin and into the skin of someone else. That way, I would be free of my present dilemma.

A few hours have passed and my family is ready to go home. I wish I could more emphatically express my love to them. I just feel so overwhelmed by my own sense of self-pity that it is difficult to do anything else. Yes, the boredom sank to a new low! I guess I will meditate and hopefully drift off into a sound sleep. Good night.

Each day brings a new chance to succeed;
Wake up, and half of the battle is won.

DAY FOURTEEN

❖❖❖❖

Today I awoke without any recollection of a dream. The Valium I received last night allowed me to sleep fairly well, and I awoke without grogginess. I am still experiencing the overwhelming sense of malaise. I perform my breathing exercises and think positive thoughts. My breakfast arrives and sits for approximately an hour. I force down a hash brown, 3/4 of a sausage, 4 ozs of orange juice, and 6 ozs of water. I eat 2 crackers to alleviate the nausea. I am growing increasingly happy about having only 7 days left in the hospital. I have made about 5 trips to the bathroom since 6:30 a.m. It is now 10:50 a.m. I remember that my period is due today, and I am faced with a strange but calming sense of knowing it will probably never come again. Thank God for my 2 children.

I could eat only 1 spoonful of my lunch. About an hour after lunch, I was informed that I needed a blood transfusion. The transfusion was to take approximately 2 hours long. I prepare for the transfusion with a shot of

Benadryl and 2 Tylenol® tablets to prevent allergic reaction and fever. I calmly await the blood. I am hoping the transfusion would eliminate the malaise. It did not happen as I hoped.

Hubby and children came to visit while I rested. We talked for awhile and the children played with creative arts packets left by a hospital volunteer. They drew pictures for me. I must have dozed off because when I looked up at the clock at 10:30 p.m., my family was gone. I wish they had awakened me to say “good night”.

❖❖❖❖

Out of a window, I see a large clock;
Time, I think to myself;
We have so little, yet so much of it;
Life is a never-ending series of ticks and tocks.

❖❖❖❖

DAY FIFTEEN

❖❖❖❖

Today I awoke feeling fairly well. I did not experience nausea and I was not groggy. There was always that question in the back of my mind about when it would start to happen. I need to receive platelets today. It is a simple process. The platelets go through my intravenous line. It is painless and the platelets enable my blood to clot at a normal rate. I really do not like taking the Benadryl because it imposes an unnatural daytime sleep upon me and causes me to stay awake at night. Being awake most of the night with nausea is the worst of things to happen.

I am thinking, I have got to be more positive about the situation. I only have six days left to go, but the doctors do not seem convinced that I will be leaving at that time. My white cell count has to be at a certain level for at least twenty-four hours before I can be released. I feel confident that I will be able to leave soon. I do not feel like eating, so I skip breakfast and lunch. Suddenly, I become famished shortly before dinner. I ate everything on my plate. It was a positive feeling for me to have an appetite again. I am expecting 2 girlfriends to visit for a sleepover today. I am sure this event will break the seemingly endless monotonous routine of being alone all night. My girlfriends along with my brother, husband and children arrived and I had a good time. If one is strong enough, a sleepover is a good remedy for stress reduction during a long hospital stay. My girlfriends and I talked and prayed. The experience was very uplifting. It allowed me to forget my overwhelming situation for a while. I would recommend a sleepover to anyone.

❖❖❖❖

When I look into myself;
I see a flame;
Wanting to burn strong and high;
But the winds and the rains;
Want to extinguish the fire;
Then, along comes oxygen;
And the fire strengthens;
And I know there will be;
And eternal glow;
Inside of me.

❖❖❖❖

DAY SIXTEEN

❖❖❖❖

I awoke feeling a bit depressed today. I guess I was sad to see my two friends leave, as they had to go to work. The nausea is gnawing at my gut. I try to think positive, but cannot help the increasing anxiety. I am ready to go home now, but I know it would be very dangerous to leave. I must be patient. I believe positive thinking will assist in a speedy recovery. I begin my daily routine of turning on the television and watching a few shows. I shower, and take a walk around the unit. I once again alternate from bed to chair, and back again. I make another attempt at drawing. This time, I painted it and it looked much better. Quite good, at least for an amateur, if I must say so myself. After a few hours, I receive a few visitors. I begin to feel a bit overheated and want to have the air conditioning turned up. In reality, I think I was subconsciously apprehensive about having so many people in the room at the same time. I am not sure what bothered me about it, but it definitely overwhelmed me. My visitors left after a couple of hours and I felt relieved. I really enjoyed seeing them, but I think I was afraid of possibly catching a germ. It seems strange that I am lonely when no one is in the room with me, but I get a little stressed when people *are* in the room with me. I think I am starting to develop symptoms of anxiety. I suspect that when one goes through a transformation of this sort, anxiety is to be expected. Go figure!

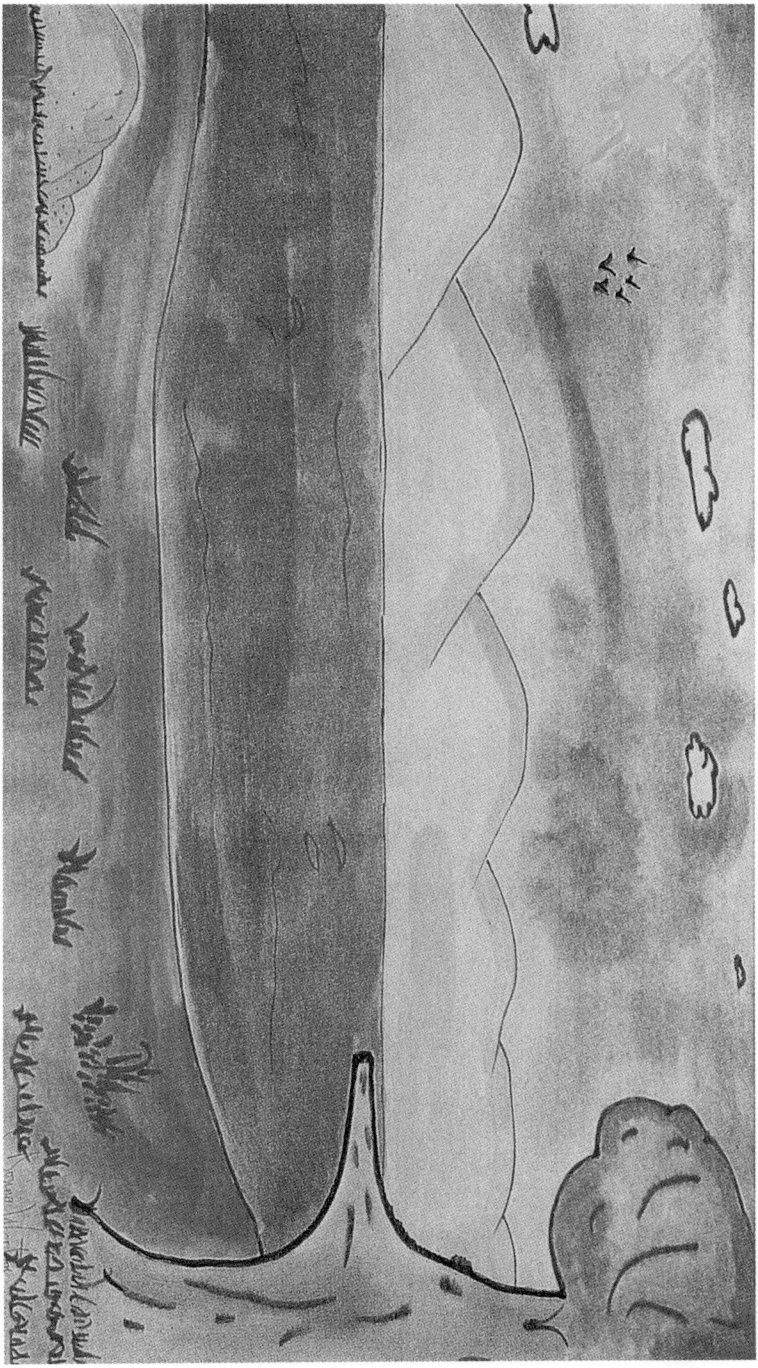

❖❖❖❖

Of all the things that I am;
A mother;
A wife;
A daughter;
A grand daughter;
A niece;
A cousin;
A friend;
A businesswoman;
A writer;
A poet;
An ambassadress;
I love being ***me*** *the most.*

❖❖❖❖

DAY SEVENTEEN

❖❖❖❖

Today I attempted to awake with a positive attitude. Unfortunately that seems to disappear when I cannot get any definite answers regarding my health from the doctors. Doctors always seem to be so general. I absolutely could not get a firm date on when I would be released from the hospital. I tried to make a determination for myself by rationalizing I did not have a fever and I did not feel weak. I figured since these two symptoms were expected, and I exhibited neither, I must be doing great and would surely be due to leave soon. I continue on with my daily routine. I wished I could go out for a walk but I know that is not possible. It is a challenge to find something new to write about every day when you are on the same boring routine. Pretty soon I will have to start telling jokes to fill the pages of this book.

The nausea has not yet subsided. I will relish the day it stops. It is almost becoming difficult to picture myself strong and vibrant again. My hair is beginning to fall out again. Losing my hair distresses me because I was ready to wear it outside without a wig or a hat. It is summer and it is a little too hot for wigs, but I feel self-conscious about going out bald. What's a girl to do? By the way, I cleaned my room today. That was a big plus.

No hair;
No brows;
Bad test;
No breast;
But that's O.K.;
Cause I'm still blessed.

DAY EIGHTEEN

❖❖❖❖

Well, it is getting closer to my scheduled time to check out of the hospital. I can almost see the light at the end of the tunnel. I am beginning to feel positive about going home. I am still nauseated, but somehow it is becoming more tolerable. I will listen to my inspirational tapes today. It looks a little rainy outside so I may sleep a little longer than usual. I have to get platelets today. I need Benadryl and Tylenol® tablets before receiving the platelets, and again, I have a vomiting episode as a result of receiving the Benadryl. I really do not like that stuff. The nurse administers Ativan, and I immediately calm down. I proceed with the platelet transfusion. The procedure went smoothly after receiving the Ativan. The day progressed relatively smoothly. I can no longer eat the hospital food. One of my cousins prepared a home cooked meal for me and brought it to me. I enjoyed it, and felt satisfied with a meal for the first time in a long time since the beginning of my hospital stay. Hubby and children were there. The children participated in their normal brother-sister routine. The time passed along without many incidents. We talked, watched television, and looked out of the window. A few hours later my family left. I watched a little more television and retired for the evening.

❖❖❖❖

In my search to find peace;
I found strength.
In my search to find joy;
I found trust.
In my search to find freedom;
I found the deep waters blue.
In my search to find love;
I found you.

This ponderance is dedicated to my husband.

❖❖❖❖

DAY NINETEEN

❖❖❖❖

Today I am thrilled to find out that my white blood cell level is .97 percent. In order to leave the hospital; I need at least a 1.0 percent white blood cell count. Even though I am on the verge of leaving very soon, I do not feel very well. My ill feelings both scare, and depress me. I feel as though I cannot afford to get sick at this stage of the medical process. I pray that I will overcome this feeling. I have body aches and I feel feverish. I develop a fever in the middle of the day and must endure a serious of blood and urine tests. I will not know the results until tomorrow. I really hope it is nothing major. I take two Tylenol® tablets to break the fever and try to rest.

After an hour or so, the fever breaks. I still do not feel the greatest, but it is tolerable. I am hoping that my white blood cell count does not decrease. My husband and children come to visit in the evening and I feel a little better. It is always good to have them around. I am starting to drink more fluids now without discomfort to my stomach. I watch television, then I focus on the growth of my white blood cells. I feel that positive imaging will aid in the increase of my white blood cell count. I do a few meditation and breathing exercises and head off to dream land. Good night!

Hope is...

__H__aving the will to
__O__verlook the odds, even when
__P__opular opinion is opposing
__E__xcessively

DAY TWENTY

❖❖❖❖

Well, as a result of focusing on my white blood cell growth, they jumped from .97 percent to 4.04 percent. Unfortunately, 4.04 is not realistic, and in most cases, drops back down within twenty-four hours. The doctors told me to expect a large increase in the white blood cell count, and then a sharp drop in the numbers. The good news is that, once that phenomenon occurs, the white blood cell count steadily increases, thereby, affording an individual a normal immune system, in time. I developed a slight fever overnight but fever medication remedied the problem. I awoke this morning with a normal temperature and slight headache. I feel quite depressed, but I am trying to gain positive spirit. It is time to pull out the gospel and the seashore music again.

Although I was expecting to leave the hospital tomorrow, the doctors say it looks more like the end of the week. I guess I can endure a few more days if that is what is best for my health. So, I sit. I wait. I hope. I pray.

Hubby and children come to visit. It is going to be a challenge to interact with the children when I get back home because they are so rambunctious, I mean, vivacious (smile). I am glad to see that I can still have a sense of humor amidst this difficult situation. I watch television with the family. I have no appetite today. So far, I have lost nineteen pounds. The weight loss is ironic, given the massive amounts of intravenous fluids flowing through my system. My family leaves for the day and I try to rest.

❖❖❖❖

I love it when I'm at the beach;
It seems as though nothing is out of reach;
The salty aroma, the crispy air;
The sounds of the seagulls as I lounge in my chair;
The feel of the breeze as it flows through my hair;
Oh wait, I forgot, I don't have any there;
O.k., so the breeze just brushes my head;
I could bring up a point, but it's better unsaid;
The sounds of waves as they rush to the shore;
I can think of few things that please me more;
Than the blue skies above the white puffy clouds;
Somehow, I don't miss the city, and the crowds;
So I'll sit and relax, and enjoy my retreat;
And I shall take in this moment until next we meet.

❖❖❖❖

DAY TWENTY ONE

❖❖❖❖

Today is my twenty-first day in the hospital. I awake groggy, but am planning to attempt to fool the doctors into thinking I am feeling better than I really feel. I do not have a fever today. Yaaah! Although I am excited about going home soon, I am also apprehensive. I suspect the ambivalence I am experiencing to be normal. I will no longer be under the watchful eyes of the doctors and nurses on the hospital staff. I feel as though my safety net will be removed. All types of thoughts are going through my mind. I have not been out of doors in close to a month. It will be different going outside again. This experience has forced me to look at life from a very different perspective. I think about the infinite amount of germs floating around in our environment. I think about how germs can so easily have a devastating effect on a compromised immune system. I think about the importance of keeping our bodies strong and fit. It is a paradox to me that during the weakest physical point in my post-birth body, to date, I am immersing myself in thoughts of the importance of a strong, healthy body.

When I get through this ordeal, I will try to eat better and exercise more.

I involve myself in the daily routine of praying, watching television, talking on the phone briefly, and looking out of the window. I pictured myself walking through those front doors. A smile covers my face. I also walked around the hospital unit. I hope this is the last time I will need to see the unit under in-patient circumstances. My heart races, excitement fills my senses. I cannot wait to go home. I corner the doctors into saying that I can go home on Thursday if I do not get a fever. It is all down hill from here.

The family comes to visit. I am happy to see them, and suddenly I am seeing the children in a new light. I see them as refreshing and spirited, instead of whiney and challenging, even though I love them just the same. The children and I draw pictures together, watch television for a short while, and the family goes home. It is difficult for me to sleep tonight in my excitement over going home soon. I will have a long session of thankful prayers.

❖❖❖❖

My soul is like ice;
Cold from the frigid air of life;
Yet my heart is warm;
Toasted by the touch of twenty little fingers;
That belongs to the hands of my children.

❖❖❖❖

DAY TWENTY TWO

❖❖❖❖

Today is Wednesday, or "hump" day, for me in more ways than one. Not only is it the middle of the week, it is the day before I go home from the hospital (provided I do not develop a fever). So, for me, that will be two humps. My bloods are good. I am poised for release. The doctors still will not totally commit to a definite release date, but I feel assured that I will be leaving tomorrow. I think about what it will feel like to wear real clothes again. I never expected the thought of putting on a pair of sweat pants to feel so good. My excitement is increasing by the hour. As I sit up in by hospital bed, filled with excitement, I begin to cry. It is a strange feeling though. I am happy for the first time in a long time but, simultaneously, I feel sad. One might argue that it is impossible to feel both extremely happy and extremely sad at the same time, but that is what I feel. Again, it is very strange. A nurse walked into the room as I sat there, and asked me why I was crying. My reply was that it was because I was going home. She looked at me strangely because even though I looked sad, I spoke happy words. That event reflected the general feeling of the moment – weird! I guess my body will go through a lot of weird stuff.

The family came. We did our usual thing and they left. I prepared my things for departure. I also gave thanks to all of the nurses on the night staff who I did not expect to see the next evening. I will go to bed tonight eager with anticipation of going home. So far, still no fever. Yaaah again!

❖❖❖❖

Bittersweet is the mood of the day;
Like the salmon, swimming upstream;
As the frolic in May
Or the little African boy on his ceremonious day;
Or the little girl, when she first sees her red;
She knows ***not*** *what lies ahead;*
The pain, the suffering, to make the world grow;
If I knew back then, today what I know;
I would brace myself;
In an effort to stay,
because;
Bittersweet is the mood of the day.

❖❖❖❖

DAY TWENTY THREE

❖❖❖❖

The day has arrived! I know I am going home today. I can just feel it in my bones. One of the doctors even alluded to it this morning during rounds. I am ready to go! The only person I want to see besides my husband, is the doctor who will remove the catheter from my chest. I receive word that they will be up shortly to remove it. I am so excited about going home; I can hardly contain myself. It is a beautiful, sunny day. I watch as the people stroll in and out of the hospital entrance. I know that within hours, one of the people will be me. I seem to have so much energy today. I wonder why (smile). I am unable to eat in all of the excitement of preparing to go home. It is mid-morning and the doctor arrives to remove my catheter. The procedure only takes about fifteen minutes. It is much easier to be removed, than to be placed. The feeling of being freed from the entourage of intravenous medications is indescribable. I almost feel as though I can fly like a bird. I can not stop smiling. Finally, a shower without tubes hanging out of my chest! I prepare the last of my belongings, and get dressed. The soft feel of the clothes pressed up against my skin is almost like a dream come true. I truly feel reborn. It is definitely a new day! My husband called to tell me he was on his way to pick me up from the hospital. I bid farewell to the staff. I did not even wait for someone to escort me out of the hospital in a wheel chair. I left the hospital as quietly and unnoticed as I had arrived. But, while I entered a scared, apprehensive woman, I departed a new person. While my mind and body would need some time to heal, my spirit was undoubtedly refreshed and renewed. As I sit on the bench at the entrance of the hospital feeling the privileges of freedom, I await my husband and my new life.

❖❖❖❖

Oh happy day;
How I must say;
How pleased I am;
To see my way;
Through trials and turmoil;
To better health;
To renewed strength;
To spiritual wealth;
To a loving family;
Who was by my side;
And never stepped off the turbulent ride;
Through thick and thin, they were right there;
Without complaint, and not a care;
My daughter, my son, my husband too;
Thank you, thank you;
I love you.

❖❖❖❖

THE DAY AFTER

❖❖❖❖

It is 7:00 a.m., and I awake to the familiarity of my home surroundings. The sun is shining brightly, and I am happy to be home. My apartment is very quiet. My husband and the children are asleep. I tiptoe through the apartment from room to room. I watch them all as they sleep peacefully. I am thankful that I can again watch my family as they slumber. I know that somewhere in the back of my mind I am wondering what the future holds for me, but right now, I am just happy to be alive. It is emotionally difficult for me to mentally revisit my hospital experience at this time. But, I think it is all right because it is not necessary to do it right now. I am happy with looking to the future. I will work towards getting stronger and healthier, both physically and mentally.

As I rode home yesterday, I admired the city and its inhabitants as they scuffled about, and I contemplated life as it passed before me in the car. I applied the experience of the car ride to how life could be if I did not take control. It would pass me by. I know that I have a lot to give to society given my interests, talents and qualifications. I have not yet finished with the world. And, I do not think the world is finished with me. I shall look out at life through an optimistic window, and cherish each moment that passes. If I am reborn, let me be renewed. I wish to share my new self with the world. If I should one day look up and find that I am physically no longer of this earth, I want to know that I have helped someone. Perhaps that someone is you. Thank you for sharing my experience with me. All blessings to you!

❖❖❖❖

See clearly;
Speak soundly;
Know fearlessly;
Love unconditionally.

❖❖❖❖

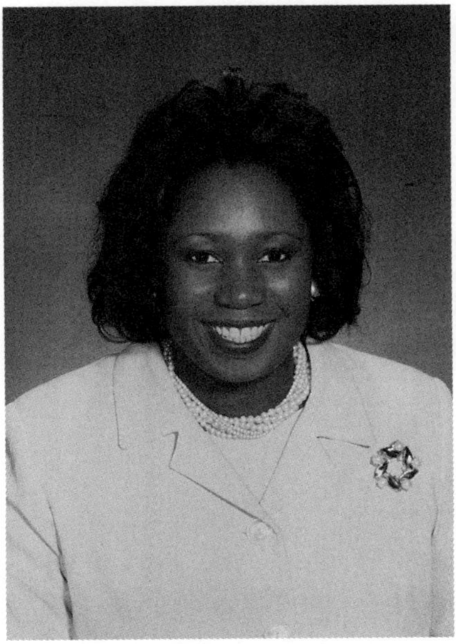

About the Author

❖❖❖❖

Donna M. Weston is a native New Yorker. She is married, and has two children. Donna devotes her time to numerous causes. She is a child advocate and is active in her community. Her liberal arts bachelor's degree, with disciplines in communications and business, enables her to do what she really loves – effectively communicate through various genres. Her flexibility allows her to work for a major accounting firm, while maintaining her own marketing and advertising home-based business. She has traveled the world, and loves people. She also plans to speak to groups about cancer survivorship.

For **questions** or **comments**, contact **Weston Enterprises**
at P.O. Box 969, New York, New York 10027
(646) 698-0941
e-mail us at: www.cellrebirth.com

To **order** this book **by phone** call:
(800) 537-6727

or **fax order requests** to:
(419)589-4040

Secure Internet order requests to:
http://www.atlasbooks.com

This book was printed by BookMasters, Inc.